https:/ fix-your-fitness.com/

Paperback ISBN: 9798870445267

Icy Resilience
Mastering Ice Baths for Enhanced Athletic Performance

CK Fix Your Fitness

KFT Publishing

Contents

Chapter 1
The Science Behind Ice Baths

Research has shown that CWI can consistently reduce the effects of DOMS and ratings of perceived exertion (RPE). A recent systematic review and meta-analysis concluded that CWI is an effective protocol for reducing the effects of DOMS 24, 48, and 96 hours post-exercise.

Owen Walker (Science for Sport)

The Benefits of Cold Therapy

COLD THERAPY, ALSO KNOWN as cryotherapy, is a practice that involves exposing the body to extremely cold temperatures for various health benefits. In recent years, it has gained popularity among fitness enthusiasts, sportspeople, gym-goers, bodybuilders, athletes, and CrossFit enthusiasts. This subchapter, titled "The Benefits of Cold Therapy," explores how incorporating cold therapy, particularly ice baths, into your fitness routine can enhance athletic performance.

One of the primary benefits of cold therapy is reduced muscle soreness and inflammation. After an intense workout or physical activity, muscles often experience micro-tears, leading to soreness and inflammation. By immersing yourself in an ice bath, the cold temperature constricts blood vessels, reducing swelling and flushing out lactic acid. This process accelerates the recovery time, allowing athletes to bounce back quicker and train harder.

Furthermore, cold therapy promotes faster muscle recovery by increasing blood circulation. When exposed to cold temperatures, blood vessels constrict, forcing blood to circulate at a faster rate. This increased circulation delivers fresh, oxygenated blood to the muscles, aiding in the removal of waste products and supplying vital nutrients. As a result, athletes experience reduced recovery time and improved overall performance.

Cold therapy also has a positive impact on the immune system. Regular ice bath sessions have been found to increase the production of white blood cells, which play a crucial role in fighting ol infections and illnesses. This enhanced immune function not only keeps athletes healthy but also allows them to maintain a consistent training schedule.

In addition to physical benefits, cold therapy can improve mental resilience. The shock of cold water triggers the release of endorphins, the body's natural mood-enhancing chemicals. This release promotes a sense of well-being, reduces stress, and boosts mental clarity. Athletes who regularly incorporate cold therapy into their routine often report increased focus, determination, and overall mental toughness.

It is important to note that cold therapy should be approached with caution and under proper guidance. Beginners should start with shorter exposure times and gradually increase as their tolerance builds. It is also advisable to consult with a healthcare professional before incorporating cold therapy into your fitness regimen, especially if you have any pre-existing medical conditions.

In conclusion, cold therapy, particularly ice baths, offers a wide range of benefits to fitness enthusiasts, sportspeople, gym-goers, bodybuilders, athletes, and CrossFit enthusiasts. By reducing muscle soreness and inflammation, promoting faster muscle recovery, enhancing immune function, and improving mental resilience, cold therapy can significantly enhance athletic performance. However, it is essential to approach cold therapy safely and seek guidance from professionals to maximize its benefits.

How Ice Baths Affect the Body

Ice baths, also known as cold-water immersion therapy, have gained significant popularity among fitness enthusiasts, athletes, and sportspeople in recent years. In this subchapter, we will explore how ice baths affect the body, unraveling the science behind their impact on athletic performance and recovery.

When subjected to an ice bath, the body's response is immediate and profound. The sudden exposure to cold water causes blood vessels to constrict, reducing blood ow to the extremities and redirecting it to vital organs. This vasoconstriction not only helps to numb pain but also aids in reducing inflammation and swelling, making ice baths a powerful tool for post-workout recovery.

Moreover, the cold temperature of the water stimulates the body's natural response to cold stress, activating the sympathetic nervous system. This activation triggers the release of adrenaline and noradrenaline, hormones that increase heart rate and blood pressure, boosting overall alertness and mental focus. Thus, ice baths not only aid physical recovery but also enhance mental resilience, making them an invaluable asset in any athlete's training regimen.

Ice baths also play a crucial role in reducing muscle soreness and improving muscle repair. The intense cold exposure promotes the release of endorphins, providing a natural analgesic effect that alleviates muscle pain. Additionally, the cold water helps remove waste products such as lactic acid, which accumulate during intense exercise, further reducing muscle soreness and enhancing recovery.

Furthermore, ice baths hav been shown to improve the body's ability to adapt to stress. Cold-water immersion stimulates the production of heat-shock proteins, which are responsible for repairing damaged cells and tissues. This adaptive response not only aids in recovery but also enhances the body's resilience to future stressors, allowing for better performance over time.

While ice baths offer numerous benefits, it is important to note that they should be used with caution and under proper guidance. It is recommended to gradually increase exposure time and temperature to avoid potential adverse effects, such as hypothermia or skin damage. Consulting with a healthcare professional or sports therapist is advisable to ensure safe and eIective implementation.

Ice baths have a profound impact on the body, enhancing athletic performance and accelerating recovery. From reducing inflammation and muscle soreness to improving mental focus and resilience, cold-water immersion therapy is a valuable tool for fitness enthusiasts, athletes, and sportspeople looking to optimize their training regimen. By mastering the art of ice baths, individuals can unlock their icy resilience and take their fitness journey to new heights.

The Role of Inflammation in Athletic Recovery

In the pursuit of peak fitness and enhanced athletic performance, athletes and fitness enthusiasts are always on the lookout for innovative techniques and strategies to aid in their recovery process. One such technique that has gained significant popularity in recent years is the use of ice baths, also known as cryotherapy or icy therapy. In this subchapter, we will explore the role of inflammation in athletic recovery and how icy therapy can effectively manage and harness its benefits.

Inflammation is a natural response of the body to injury or intense physical activity. When we engage in strenuous exercise, microscopic damage occurs in our muscles, resulting in inflammation. While inflammation is a necessary part of the healing process, excessive or prolonged inflammation can hinder recovery and hinder performance. This is where icy therapy comes into play.

Icy therapy, specifically ice baths, involves immersing oneself in cold water for a specific duration, typically between 10 to 15 minutes. The cold temperature constricts blood vessels, reducing blood flow to the affected area. As a result, inflammation is effectively controlled, minimizing the extent of tissue damage and speeding up the recovery process.

By reducing inflammation, ice baths help athletes and fitness enthusiasts recover faster from intense workouts or competitions. The cold immersion also helps alleviate muscle soreness and stiffness, allowing individuals to bounce back quickly for their next training session. Additionally, icy therapy promotes the removal of waste products, such as lactic acid, from the muscles, further aiding in the recovery process.

However, it is important to note that icy therapy should be used in conjunction with other recovery strategies, such as proper nutrition, adequate rest, and targeted stretching and mobility exercises. Ice baths should be used as a complementary tool to enhance recovery, rather than a standalone solution.

For fitness enthusiasts, sportspeople, gym-goers, bodybuilders, athletes, and cross-fit enthusiasts seeking to optimize their recovery and maximize their performance, understanding the role of inflammation in athletic recovery is crucial. Incorporating icy therapy, such as ice baths, into their recovery routine can provide them with a competitive edge by reducing inflammation, promoting faster recovery, and ultimately enhancing their overall athletic performance.

In the following chapters, we will delve deeper into the art of ice baths, exploring techniques for optimal immersion, duration, and temperature, as well as tips for maximizing the benefits of icy therapy. Get ready to master the art of ice baths and unlock your icy resilience for peak fitness!

Chapter 2
Preparing for an Ice Bath

"Give me six hours to chop down a tree and I will
spend the first four sharpening the axe."

Abraham Lincoln

Understanding the Basics of Cold Exposure

I N THE JOURNEY TO achieve peak fitness, athletes and fitness
enthusiasts are constantly seeking new and innovative ways to
enhance their performance and recovery. One such method that
has gained significant attention in recent years is cold exposure,
particularly through the practice of ice baths. In this subchapter, we
will delve into the basics of cold exposure and how it can be harnessed
to unlock the full potential of your athletic abilities.

Cold exposure, also known as cryotherapy, involves subjecting the body to extreme cold temperatures for a specific duration. This can be achieved through various methods, including ice baths, cold showers, or specialized cryotherapy chambers. The fundamental principle behind cold exposure lies in its ability to induce physiological adaptations that promote improved athletic performance and recovery.

When exposed to cold temperatures, the body triggers a series of physiological responses to maintain internal homeostasis. One of the key mechanisms is vasoconstriction, where blood vessels narrow to reduce blood ow to the extremities in order to preserve core body temperature. This process aids in reducing in ammation and swelling, which is particularly beneficial for athletes recovering from intense training sessions or injuries.

Another crucial adaptation resulting from cold exposure is the activation of brown adipose tissue (BAT), commonly known as brown fat. Unlike white fat, which stores energy, BAT generates heat by burning calories. By activating and increasing the amount of brown fat in the body, individuals can enhance their metabolic rate and potentially reduce body fat percentage.

Cold exposure also stimulates the release of endorphins, known as the body's natural painkillers and mood enhancers. This can lead to an improved sense of well-being and mental resilience, which is vital for athletes during intense training or competitions.

Incorporating cold exposure into your fitness routine requires careful planning and gradual adaptation. Starting with shorter exposure times and gradually increasing the duration and intensity is recommended to avoid potential adverse elects. It is crucial to consult with a healthcare professional or a qualified coach who can guide you through the process and ensure your safety.

By understanding the basics of cold exposure, you can harness its potential to unlock enhanced athletic performance and recovery. Whether you are a professional athlete, a gym-goer, or a fitness enthusiast, incorporating cold exposure techniques such as ice baths into your routine can provide a competitive edge and help you reach your fitness goals. So, embrace the icy resilience and embark on a journey to master the art of ice baths for peak fitness.

Setting Up the Perfect Ice Bath Environment

Creating the ideal ice bath environment is crucial for maximizing the benefits of this powerful recovery technique. In this book we delve into the art of setting up the perfect ice bath environment to help fitness enthusiasts, sportspeople, gym-goers, bodybuilders, athletes, and CrossFit enthusiasts achieve peak fitness through icy therapy.

The first step in setting up your ice bath environment is finding the right location. Ideally, choose a quiet and private space where you can fully immerse yourself in the experience without distractions. A bathroom, basement, or even a dedicated ice bath room can serve as a suitable location. Ensure the space is well- ventilated to prevent excessive humidity and ensure a comfortable experience.

Next, consider the temperature of the water. The optimal temperature for an ice bath is between 50 to 59 degrees Fahrenheit (10 to 15 degrees Celsius). Use a reliable thermometer to monitor the water temperature accurately. It's important to maintain consistency in temperature to achieve the desired therapeutic effects. Consider using a thermometer that can be submerged in the water to ensure precise measurements.

Another essential aspect of the perfect ice bath environment is the addition of ice or cold packs. Adding ice helps to lower the water temperature and intensify the eIects of the therapy. Use large bags of ice or ice packs to cool the water effectively. Monitor the temperature regularly, adding or removing ice as needed to maintain the desired range.

To enhance the ambiance and create a relaxing atmosphere, consider incorporating soothing elements. Soft lighting, calming music, or even scented candles can help create a serene and enjoyable experience. These elements can also contribute to a positive mindset, making the ice bath more mentally and emotionally rejuvenating.

Finally, it is crucial to prioritize safety when setting up the ice bath environment. Ensure the bath is stable and secure, with non-slip mats or grips to prevent accidents. Have a timer or stopwatch nearby to monitor your time accurately and prevent overexposure. Always have a towel, robe, or warm clothing readily available to cozy up in after the ice bath.

Setting up the perfect ice bath environment is essential to harness the full potential of icy therapy. By finding the right location, monitoring the water temperature, incorporating ice, creating a serene ambiance, and prioritizing safety, you can enhance your ice bath experience and reap the benefits of improved athletic performance and faster recovery. Take the plunge into icy resilience and master the art of ice baths for peak fitness!

Mental Preparation Techniques

In the quest to achieve peak fitness and enhance athletic performance, mental preparation techniques play a crucial role. In this subchapter, we will explore the various strategies that can help you develop icy resilience through mastering the art of ice baths. These techniques are not just limited to professional athletes, but are equally beneficial for fitness enthusiasts, sportspeople, gym-goers, bodybuilders, athletes, and cross fitters.

1. Visualization: Visualizing success is a powerful tool that can boost your mental strength and endurance. Before stepping into an ice bath, close your eyes and imagine yourself handling the intense cold with ease. Visualize the benefits it will bring to your body and the feeling of accomplishment afterwards. This technique will help you build confidence and reduce anxiety.

2. Breath Control: Deep breathing exercises can help you manage the discomfort and stress associated with ice baths. Practice diaphragmatic breathing, inhaling deeply through your nose and exhaling slowly through your mouth. Focusing on your breath will not only regulate your body's response to the cold but also calm your mind.

3. Positive Affirmations: Affirmations are positive statements that can reprogram your mindset and boost your confidence. Repeat affirmations such as "I am strong," "I am resilient," or "I embrace challenges" before and during your ice bath. These affirmations will reinforce your mental strength and help you push through any discomfort.

4. Mindfulness: Being present in the moment is crucial during an ice bath. Instead of resisting the cold, embrace it. Pay attention to the sensations in your body, observe your thoughts without judgment, and focus on the present experience. Practicing mindfulness will help you develop mental resilience and enhance your ability to tolerate discomfort.

5. Goal Setting: Setting clear goals for your ice bath sessions can help you stay motivated and focused. Whether it's increasing your bath duration, improving your mental endurance, or reducing your recovery time, having specific objectives will give you something to strive for. Celebrate your achievements along the way to maintain a positive mindset.

By incorporating these mental preparation techniques into your ice bath routine, you will not only enhance your physical performance but also strengthen your mental toughness. Remember, icy resilience is not just about enduring the cold; it's about training your mind to overcome challenges and achieve your fitness goals. Embrace the power of mental preparation, and unlock your full potential in the realm of icy therapy.

Chapter 3

Getting Started with Ice Baths

"The secret of getting ahead is getting started."

Mark Twain

Gradual Exposure to Cold

IN THE QUEST FOR peak fitness, athletes and fitness enthusiasts are constantly seeking innovative methods to enhance their performance and recovery. One such method that has gained significant attention in recent years is the practice of icy therapy, specifically ice baths. The section delves into the importance of acclimating your body to cold temperatures gradually.

Ice baths have been used for centuries to aid recovery, reduce inflammation, and improve overall well-being. However, diving straight into icy water without proper preparation can do more harm than good. That's where gradual exposure to cold comes into play.

For fitness enthusiasts, sportspeople, gym-goers, bodybuilders, athletes, and CrossFit enthusiasts, it is crucial to understand the various stages involved in acclimating your body to cold temperatures. This process ensures that your body adapts to the cold gradually, minimizing the risk of shock or injury.

We provide a detailed roadmap on how to gradually expose your body to cold water immersion. We start by explaining the initial steps, which involve using cold showers or alternating hot and cold showers to familiarize your body with temperature changes. This technique helps to improve blood circulation, strengthen the immune system, and increase the body's tolerance to cold.

As you progress, we guide you through the next phase, introducing ice packs or ice baths for short durations. We emphasize the importance of listening to your body and gradually increasing exposure time as you become more comfortable. This gradual approach allows your body to adapt and reap the full benefits of icy therapy.

Moreover, we share essential tips on managing discomfort, such as breathing techniques and mental preparation strategies. These techniques will help you stay focused and develop mental resilience while undergoing cold exposure.

By following the principles outlined in this subchapter, you will master the art of gradual exposure to cold, ultimately enabling you to unlock the full potential of icy therapy for peak fitness. Whether you are an athlete aiming to enhance performance or a fitness enthusiast seeking faster recovery, this subchapter will serve as a comprehensive guide to safely and effectively incorporate icy therapy into your routine.

"Icy Resilience: Mastering Ice Baths for Enhanced Athletic Performance" is your ultimate resource to understand the science behind ice baths, learn practical techniques, and explore the vast benefits of icy therapy. Embrace the power of gradual exposure to cold, and unlock your true potential.

The Ideal Temperature for Ice Baths

When it comes to ice baths, one of the most important factors to consider is the temperature of the water. The ideal temperature can greatly impact the effectiveness and benefit of this icy therapy. In this subchapter, we will delve into the science behind finding the perfect temperature for your ice baths.

For fitness enthusiasts, sports people, gym-goers, bodybuilders, athletes, and cross fitters, ice baths have become a popular method for enhancing athletic performance and aiding recovery. The proper temperature can make all the difference in reaping the desired benefits.

Research suggests that the ideal temperature for ice baths falls within the range of 10 to 15 degrees Celsius (50 to 59 degrees Fahrenheit). This temperature range allows for optimal cooling of the body without causing excessive discomfort or potential harm. Lower temperatures may be too cold for most individuals, leading to prolonged discomfort and potential tissue damage.

The key to finding the right temperature lies in understanding the physiological response of the body to cold exposure. When immersed in cold water, blood vessels constrict, reducing blood ow to the extremities and diverting it to the core. This vasoconstriction helps to reduce inflammation and minimize tissue damage caused by intense workouts or injuries.

At temperatures around 10 to 15 degrees Celsius, the body triggers a physiological response known as cold- induced thermogenesis. This response activates brown adipose tissue, which generates heat to keep the body warm. As a result, the body burns more calories, aiding in weight loss and promoting overall fitness.

It is important to note that individual tolerance and personal preference play a significant role in determining the ideal temperature for ice baths. Some individuals may prefer slightly colder temperatures, finding them more invigorating, while others may opt for a slightly warmer experience.

Experimentation is key when determining the optimal temperature for your ice baths. Start with temperatures around 10 to 15 degrees Celsius (50 to 59 degrees Fahrenheit) and gradually adjust according to your comfort level and desired effects. Keep in mind that the purpose of an ice bath is to stimulate and rejuvenate, not to cause pain or discomfort.

In summary, the ideal temperature for ice baths falls within the range of 10 to15 degrees Celsius (50 to 59 degrees Fahrenheit). This temperature allows for effective cooling, vasoconstriction, and the activation of cold-induced thermogenesis. Experimentation and personal preference should guide you in finding the perfect temperature that maximizes the benefits of ice baths while keeping you motivated on your fitness journey.

Recommended Duration for Ice Baths

In the world of fitness and sports performance, athletes are always seeking new ways to enhance their physical abilities and gain a competitive edge. One method that has gained significant popularity in recent years is the use of ice baths. These cold-water immersions have been shown to provide numerous benefits, including faster recovery, reduced muscle soreness, and improved overall performance. However, it is essential to understand that the duration of an ice bath plays a crucial role in maximizing its benefits.

When it comes to the recommended duration for ice baths, there is no one-size-fits-all answer. The duration can vary depending on factors such as the individual's fitness level, the intensity of their training, and their specific goals. Nevertheless, there are some general guidelines that can help fitness enthusiasts, sportspeople, gym-goers, bodybuilders, athletes, and cross fitters determine the optimal duration for their ice bath sessions.

For most individuals, a typical ice bath duration ranges from 10 to 20 minutes. During this time, the cold water works to constrict blood vessels and reduce inflammation, which aids in the recovery process. It is important to note that the first few minutes may feel uncomfortable, but as the body adjusts to the cold, the benefits become more apparent.

However, it is crucial to avoid exceeding the recommended duration, as prolonged exposure to cold temperatures can have adverse effects. Extended ice bath sessions can lead to tissue damage, increased stiffness, and even hypothermia. Therefore, it is essential to listen to your body and gradually increase the duration over time, rather than pushing yourself to extremes right from the start.

It is worth mentioning that the duration can also vary based on the specific goals of the individual. For instance, if the primary aim is to reduce muscle soreness after an intense workout, a shorter ice bath duration of around 10 minutes may suffice. On the other hand, if the focus is on enhancing recovery and reducing inflammation, a longer duration of 15 to 20 minutes might be more beneficial.

In conclusion, ice baths can be a powerful tool for enhancing athletic performance and promoting recovery. However, it is crucial to find the optimal duration that suits your individual needs and goals. By following the general guidelines mentioned above and listening to your body, you can harness the power of icy resilience and master the art of ice baths for peak fitness.

Chapter 4

Techniques for Enduring Ice Baths

"Endurance is one of the most difficult disciplines, but it is to the one who endures that the final victory comes."

Gautama Buddha

Breathing Exercises for Cold Adaptation

IN THE QUEST FOR peak fitness and enhanced athletic performance, one often ventures into uncharted territories. One such territory is the realm of ice baths, where icy cold water becomes a powerful tool for physical and mental resilience. To fully embrace the benefits of icy therapy, mastering breathing exercises for cold adaptation is an essential skill for fitness enthusiasts, sports people, gym-goers, bodybuilders, athletes, and CrossFit enthusiasts alike.

When exposed to extreme cold, our body's natural response is to contract, seeking warmth and protection. However, through specific breathing techniques, we can train our bodies to adapt to the cold, allowing us to endure longer and reap the rewards of this unique training method.

One effective breathing exercise for cold adaptation is the Wim Hof Method[1]. This technique, developed by the renowned "Iceman" Wim Hof, focuses on deep, controlled breaths to optimize oxygen intake and influence the autonomic nervous system. By practicing this method regularly, individuals can strengthen their immune system, increase energy levels, and develop a heightened ability to withstand cold temperatures.

To begin, find a comfortable seated position and take a moment to relax. Inhale deeply through your nose, filling your lungs with air, and then exhale slowly through your mouth. Continue this controlled breathing pattern for several minutes, focusing on the sensation of the breath entering and leaving your body. Gradually increase the duration of your inhales and exhales, allowing your breath to become slower and deeper with each repetition.

As you become more comfortable with this technique, you can experiment with adding breath holds at the end of your exhales. This practice mimics the body's response to cold exposure, training it to remain calm and composed even in freezing conditions. Start by holding your breath for a few seconds, gradually increasing the

---

1. https://www.wimhofmethod.com/practice-the-method

duration as your body adapts. Remember to always listen to your body and never push yourself beyond your limits.

Incorporating breathing exercises for cold adaptation into your routine will not only enhance your ice bath experiences but also improve your overall physical and mental resilience. As you continue to practice and develop your cold adaptation skills, you will unlock new levels of performance, pushing your limits and achieving new athletic heights.

So, whether you're a seasoned athlete or just starting your fitness journey, mastering breathing exercises for cold adaptation is a valuable skill worth exploring. Embrace the icy resilience that comes with ice baths and unleash your full potential in the world of fitness and sports.

Visualization and Mental Techniques

In the pursuit of peak fitness, athletes and fitness enthusiasts often focus solely on physical training and neglect the crucial role of mental preparation. However, in recent years, there has been a growing recognition of the power of visualization and mental techniques in enhancing athletic performance. In this subchapter, we will explore the fascinating world of visualization and provide you with practical techniques to harness its potential.

Visualization is the practice of creating vivid mental images of desired outcomes or experiences. By visualizing success, athletes can prime their minds and bodies for optimal performance. This technique has been extensively used by high-performing athletes across various sports, including bodybuilding, crossfit, and professional sports. The power of visualization lies in its ability to activate the same neural pathways as physical practice, thereby improving muscle memory and enhancing performance.

One of the most eIective visualization techniques is the creation of a mental rehearsal. This involves mentally rehearsing your performance, step by step, in your mind's eye. Whether it's a weightlifting session, a crossfit competition, or a marathon, mentally visualizing each movement and every detail of your performance can help improve coordination, focus, and overall execution.

Another powerful mental technique is the use of affirmations and positive self-talk. By repeating positive statements about yourself and your abilities, you can cultivate a confident and resilient mindset. Affirmations such as "I am strong," "I am capable," and "I am prepared" can help boost self-belief and overcome self- doubt, leading to improved performance and greater resilience.

Furthermore, visualization can be combined with relaxation techniques to enhance its eIectiveness. By practicing deep breathing exercises and progressive muscle relaxation, athletes can create a calm and focused mental state, which is essential for optimal visualization. These techniques can be particularly valuable in highly stressful situations, allowing athletes to maintain composure and perform at their best.

In conclusion, visualization and mental techniques are powerful tools that can significantly enhance athletic performance. By incorporating these practices into your training routine, you can tap into the untapped potential of your mind and unlock new levels of performance. Whether you are a bodybuilder, a crossfit enthusiast, or an athlete, visualization can be the missing piece to take your fitness journey to the next level. So, dare to visualize your success, and let your mind pave the way to icy resilience and peak performance.

Distraction Techniques to Manage Discomfort

When it comes to pushing your limits and achieving peak fitness, ice baths have become a popular choice among fitness enthusiasts, bodybuilders, athletes, and sportspeople. The benefits of icy therapy are well- documented, ranging from reducing in ammation and muscle soreness to enhancing recovery and performance. However, the discomfort that comes with immersing your body in freezing cold water can be quite challenging to endure. That's where distraction techniques come into play.

In this subchapter, we will explore various distraction techniques that can help you manage discomfort during your icy therapy sessions. By diverting your attention away from the cold, you can better endure the physical sensations, allowing you to reap the full benefits of ice baths for enhanced athletic performance.

One eIective distraction technique is visualization. By closing your eyes and envisioning yourself in a warm, tropical paradise, you can transport your mind away from the icy water. Imagine the sun warming your skin, the sound of waves crashing on the shore, and the sensation of sand beneath your feet. This mental escape can provide a sense of relaxation and help you power through the chilling sensation.

Another technique to consider is engaging in deep breathing exercises. Focusing on your breath can help calm your mind and relax your body, reducing the perception of discomfort. Take slow, deep breaths in through your nose, and exhale slowly through your mouth. Concentrating on your breath can serve as a powerful distraction and provide a sense of control over the situation.

Music can also be a powerful tool to distract your mind from the cold. Create a playlist of your favorite upbeat and motivational tunes that you can listen to during your icy therapy sessions. The rhythm and lyrics can help shift your focus away from the discomfort and pump you up with energy and determination.

Furthermore, engaging in conversation with a workout partner or a friend can help divert your attention. Sharing stories, discussing fitness goals, or simply engaging in light-hearted banter can create a positive and supportive environment that takes your mind oI the cold.

Experiment with these distraction techniques and find what works best for you. Remember, the discomfort experienced during ice baths is temporary, but the benefits to your athletic performance are long-lasting. By mastering the art of distraction, you can enhance your icy resilience and take your fitness journey to new heights.

Chapter 5

Maximizing Athletic Performance Through Ice Baths

"You gain strength, courage and confidence by every experience in which you really stop to look fear in the face. You must do the thing you think you cannot do"

Eleanor Roosevelt

Ice Baths for Recovery and Muscle Repair

ICE BATHS HAVE LONG been used by athletes and fitness enthusiasts as a powerful tool for enhancing recovery and promoting muscle repair. In this subchapter, we will delve into the benefits of ice baths, how to properly incorporate them into your fitness routine, and why they are a valuable addition to any athlete's training regimen.

Ice baths, also known as cold water immersion, involve submerging the body in ice-cold water for a short period of time after intense physical activity. The extreme cold causes blood vessels to constrict, reducing inflammation and swelling in the muscles and joints. This process, known as vasoconstriction, helps to flush out metabolic waste products and toxins, aiding in the recovery process.

One of the key benefits of ice baths is their ability to reduce muscle soreness and speed up the recovery time. After a grueling workout or competition, muscle fibers undergo microscopic damage. Ice baths help to minimize this damage by reducing the buildup of lactic acid and other metabolic byproducts that contribute to muscle soreness. By decreasing inflammation and swelling, ice baths also assist in preventing the onset of delayed onset muscle soreness (DOMS).

Furthermore, ice baths can improve circulation and promote the delivery of oxygen and nutrients to tired muscles. The cold temperature stimulates blood flow, which aids in the removal of metabolic waste and provides essential nutrients to promote healing and repair. This increased circulation can also help reduce the risk of muscle imbalances and injuries.

When incorporating ice baths into your fitness routine, it is essential to follow proper guidelines to ensure safety and maximize benefits. Start by gradually acclimating your body to the cold temperature by beginning with shorter durations and gradually increasing the time. Aim for a duration of 10-15 minutes in water between 10-15 degrees Celsius for optimal results. It is also recommended to consult with a healthcare professional or trainer before starting ice bath therapy, especially if you have any underlying medical conditions.

In conclusion, ice baths are a valuable tool for recovery and muscle repair for athletes, fitness enthusiasts, bodybuilders, and individuals engaged in intense physical activity. By reducing inflammation, promoting circulation, and aiding in the removal of metabolic waste, ice baths can enhance recovery time, reduce muscle soreness, and prevent injuries. Incorporating ice baths into your fitness routine can help you achieve peak performance and maintain icy resilience.

Ice Baths for Reducing Inflammation

In today's fast-paced world, fitness enthusiasts, sportspeople, gym-goers, bodybuilders, athletes, and cross fit enthusiasts are always on the lookout for innovative ways to enhance their performance and speed up recovery. One such technique gaining significant attention is the use of ice baths to reduce inflammation. In this subchapter of we will delve into the benefits and techniques of using ice baths for reducing inflammation, allowing you to optimize your recovery and push your limits further.

Inflammation is a natural response of the body to injury or intense physical activity. While it is an essential part of the healing process, excessive inflammation can hinder recovery and performance. This is where ice baths come into play. By immersing your body in cold water, typically ranging from 10 to 15 degrees Celsius (50 to 59 degrees

Fahrenheit), you can effectively reduce inflammation and promote faster recovery.

Ice baths work by constricting blood vessels, which helps to decrease blood flow and limit the release of inflammatory substances. Additionally, the cold temperature numbs the nerve endings, providing pain relief and reducing muscle soreness. This makes ice baths an excellent tool for athletes looking to bounce back quickly from intense training sessions or competitions.

To reap the benefits of ice baths for reducing inflammation, it is important to follow a few guidelines. First and foremost, consult with a healthcare professional or sports therapist to ensure ice baths are suitable for your specific needs and conditions. Start with shorter durations, around 5 to 10 minutes, and gradually increase the time as your body adapts. Always monitor your body's response and listen to any discomfort or pain signals it may send.

To enhance the effectiveness of ice baths, consider incorporating contrast therapy, alternating between cold and hot water. This method further improves blood circulation and aids in flushing out toxins from the muscles.Additionally, practicing proper breathing techniques during the ice bath can help you relax and optimize the benefits.

Remember, ice baths are just one piece of the puzzle when it comes to optimizing athletic performance and recovery. They should be used in conjunction with a well-rounded training program, proper nutrition, and adequate rest. By mastering the art of ice baths for peak fitness, you can unlock your body's full potential and achieve new heights in your athletic journey.

In summary, ice baths have emerged as a powerful tool for reducing inflammation and enhancing recovery in the world of fitness and sports. By incorporating ice baths into your routine, you can accelerate your body's healing process, alleviate muscle soreness, and optimize your overall performance. So, embrace the power of cold and take your athletic journey to new icy heights with ice baths.

Ice Baths for Improving Endurance and Stamina

Ice baths have long been used by athletes and fitness enthusiasts as a powerful tool to enhance endurance and stamina. In this subchapter, we will explore the benefits and science behind incorporating ice baths into your training routine. Whether you are a professional athlete, bodybuilder, or simply someone looking to take their fitness to the next level, understanding the power of icy resilience is essential.

Endurance and stamina are crucial components of any fitness regime. They determine how long you can push your body to perform at its best, whether you are running a marathon or lifting weights. Ice baths offer a unique approach to improving these aspects of your fitness.

When you expose your body to cold temperatures during an ice bath, it triggers a series of physiological responses. One of the key benefits is vasoconstriction, which causes blood vessels to constrict, reducing blood flow to the muscles. This temporary reduction in blood flow helps to flush out lactic acid and other metabolic waste products that accumulate during intense workouts. As a result, your muscles recover faster, allowing you to train harder and longer.

Ice baths also stimulate the production of mitochondria, the powerhouses of our cells responsible for energy production. By increasing the number of mitochondria in your muscles, ice baths can significantly enhance your endurance and stamina. This means you will be able to sustain high-intensity workouts for longer periods, giving you a competitive edge in any sport or fitness activity.

Additionally, ice baths have been shown to improve mental resilience. The cold exposure activates the sympathetic nervous system, triggering the release of endorphins and other mood-enhancing chemicals. This can help you push through mental barriers, allowing you to stay focused and motivated during challenging workouts.

It is important to note that ice baths should be approached with caution. Proper technique and guidance are essential to ensure safety and maximize benefits. Consulting with a trained professional or sports therapist is highly recommended before incorporating ice baths into your training routine.

In conclusion, ice baths are a powerful tool for improving endurance and stamina. By incorporating this icy therapy into your fitness regime, you can enhance your performance, speed up recovery, and push through mental barriers. Embrace the power of icy resilience and take your fitness journey to new heights.

Chapter 6

Combining Ice Baths with Other Recovery Methods

"You don't drown by falling in the water; you drown
by staying there."

Edwin Louis Cole

Contrast Therapy: Alternating Hot and Cold

IN THE WORLD OF fitness and athletic performance, finding ways
to enhance recovery and improve performance is crucial. One
method that has gained popularity among fitness enthusiasts, sports

people, gym-goers, bodybuilders, athletes, and cross fit enthusiasts is contrast therapy. This subchapter will delve into the concept of contrast therapy, specifically focusing on alternating hot and cold temperatures, and how it can be a game-changer for achieving peak fitness.

Contrast therapy, also known as hot-cold therapy or hot and cold immersion, involves alternating between hot and cold temperatures to stimulate the body's natural healing mechanisms. This technique has been used for centuries and has been proven to have numerous benefits for athletic performance and recovery.

The alternating hot and cold temperatures in contrast therapy help to increase circulation, reduce inflammation, and speed up recovery. When exposed to heat, blood vessels expand, allowing for improved blood flow and oxygen delivery to the muscles. This helps to flush out metabolic waste products, reduce muscle soreness, and promote tissue repair. On the other hand, cold temperatures cause blood vessels to constrict, reducing inflammation and swelling, and numbing pain receptors.

By alternating between hot and cold temperatures, the body goes through a process of vasoconstriction and vasodilation, which enhances the efficiency of the circulatory system. This process aids in reducing muscle fatigue, accelerating recovery, and improving overall athletic performance.

Contrast therapy can be applied using various methods, such as ice baths, cold showers, saunas, hot tubs, and hot packs. The duration of each temperature exposure and the number of cycles can vary depending on individual preferences and goals.

It is important to note that contrast therapy should be approached with caution and under the guidance of a qualified professional.

Gradually increasing the intensity and duration of the hot and cold stimuli is crucial to avoid any potential adverse effects.

In conclusion, contrast therapy, specifically alternating hot and cold temperatures, is a powerful tool for fitness enthusiasts, athletes, and individuals looking to take their performance to the next level. By incorporating contrast therapy into your routine, you can experience improved circulation, reduced inflammation, enhanced recovery, and ultimately, peak fitness. So, why not take the plunge and explore the world of contrast therapy to unleash your icy resilience?

Cryotherapy: Whole-Body Cold Exposure

In the quest for enhanced athletic performance, athletes and fitness enthusiasts are constantly seeking new and innovative ways to push their bodies to their limits. One technique that has gained significant attention in recent years is cryotherapy, specifically whole-body cold exposure. This section of "Icy Resilience" explores the benefits and techniques of cryotherapy and how it can be utilized to optimize athletic performance.

Cryotherapy involves exposing the body to extremely cold temperatures, typically ranging from -100 to -160 degrees Celsius, for a short period of time. This cold exposure triggers a myriad of physiological responses within the body, leading to a range of potential benefits for athletes. One of the primary advantages of cryotherapy is it ability to reduce inflammation and promote faster recovery. By subjecting the body to extreme cold, cryotherapy helps to constrict blood vessels, which can alleviate swelling and soreness, and accelerate the healing process.

Another key benefit of cryotherapy is its ability to enhance performance and endurance. By exposing the body to extreme cold, cryotherapy stimulates the release of endorphins and adrenaline, which can improve mental focus, energy levels, and overall performance. Additionally, cryotherapy has been shown to increase the production of red blood cells, which transport oxygen to the muscles, thereby improving endurance and stamina.

To effectively utilize cryotherapy, individuals can choose from various methods, including whole-body cryotherapy chambers, ice baths, or cryo-saunas. Each method has its own advantages and can be tailored to suit individual preferences. However, it is important to note that cryotherapy should always be performed under the supervision of a trained professional to ensure safety and proper technique.

For fitness enthusiasts, sportspeople, gym-goers, bodybuilders, athletes, and cross-fit enthusiasts, cryotherapy can be a valuable tool in their training arsenal. By incorporating regular cryotherapy sessions into their routine, individuals can experience faster recovery, reduced inflammation, improved endurance, and enhanced performance. However, it is crucial to understand that cryotherapy is just one aspect of a comprehensive training program, and should be used in conjunction with proper nutrition, rest, and other training methodologies.

Cryotherapy, specifically whole-body cold exposure, is a powerful technique that can significantly benefit athletes and fitness enthusiasts alike. By harnessing the power of extreme cold, individuals can optimize their athletic performance, accelerate recovery, and improve overall endurance. With proper guidance and supervision, cryotherapy can be a valuable addition to any training regimen, helping individuals achieve their fitness goals and unlock their full potential.

Compression Therapy and Ice Baths

Compression Therapy and Ice Baths are two powerful tools that can greatly enhance athletic performance and aid in post-workout recovery. In this subchapter, we will explore the benefits and techniques of these methods, providing valuable information for fitness enthusiasts, sports people, gym-goers, bodybuilders, athletes, and cross fit enthusiasts.

Compression Therapy is a technique that involves applying pressure to specific areas of the body using compression garments or wraps. This therapy is known to improve blood circulation, reduce muscle soreness, and speed up the recovery process. By compressing the muscles, it helps to flush out metabolic waste products, such as lactic acid, which contribute to muscle fatigue. Additionally, compression therapy can prevent swelling and inflammation, allowing athletes to train harder and recover faster.

Ice Baths, on the other hand, are a form of cold therapy that involves immersing the body in icy cold water. This technique has been used for centuries to relieve muscle soreness, reduce inflammation, and promote overall recovery. When exposed to cold temperatures, the blood vessels constrict, forcing metabolic waste products out of the muscles. Ice baths also help to numb the nerve endings, reducing pain and discomfort. This subchapter will provide guidance on how to properly prepare and execute an ice bath, ensuring maximum benefits and safety.

When used in combination, Compression Therapy and ice Baths an have a synergistic effect on athletic performance. Compression garments can be worn during an ice bath, further enhancing the therapeutic benefits. The compression helps to increase the rate of cooling, allowing the muscles to recover more efficiently. This subchapter will delve into the science behind this combination and oIer practical tips on how to incorporate it into your training routine.

Whether you are a professional athlete or just starting your fitness journey, understanding the benefits of Compression Therapy and Ice Baths can give you an edge in achieving your goals. By incorporating these techniques into your training regimen, you can experience reduced muscle soreness, faster recovery, and improved overall performance.

In conclusion, this subchapter serves as a comprehensive guide for fitness enthusiasts, sports people, gym- goers, bodybuilders, athletes, and cross fit enthusiasts who want to optimize their training and recovery. By mastering the art of Compression Therapy and Ice Baths, you can unlock your icy resilience and reach new heights in your athletic endeavours.

Chapter 7
Safety Precautions and Common Mistakes

"No Safety, Know Pain. Know Safety, No Pain."

Anonymous

Proper Monitoring of Body Temperature

ONE OF THE KEY aspects of mastering ice baths for enhanced athletic performance is the proper monitoring of body temperature. As fitness enthusiasts, sports people, gym-goers, bodybuilders, athletes, and cross fit enthusiasts, you understand the importance of maintaining optimal body temperature during intense physical activities. In this subchapter, we will delve into the significance of monitoring your body temperature during ice therapy to maximize its benefits.

Ice baths, also known as cold water immersion, have gained popularity in the fitness world due to their numerous benefits. These include reducing muscle inflammation, speeding up recovery, improving circulation, and boosting overall athletic performance. However, without proper monitoring, there is a risk of overexposure to cold temperatures, which can have adverse effects on your body.

To ensure the safe and effective use of ice baths, it is crucial to monitor your body temperature throughout the process. This can be done using various methods, such as using a digital thermometer or wearable temperature sensors. By regularly checking your body temperature, you can ensure that it remains within a safe and optimal range.

During an ice bath session, your body will naturally start to cool down as it is exposed to the cold water. However, it is essential to avoid prolonged exposure that can lead to hypothermia or other cold-related injuries. By monitoring your body temperature, you can determine the ideal duration for your ice bath session.

Additionally, monitoring your body temperature can help you gauge your body's response to the ice bath. If your temperature drops too quickly or remains low even after the session, it may indicate that your body is struggling to regulate its temperature. This information can help you adjust the duration or intensity of your ice bath sessions accordingly.

Furthermore, monitoring your body temperature is crucial for avoiding overheating during the rewarming process. After an ice bath, your body will naturally warm up to restore its core temperature.

However, if this process occurs too rapidly or if your body temperature rises above normal levels, it can lead to discomfort or even thermal stress. By closely monitoring your body temperature during the rewarming phase, you can ensure a safe and gradual return to normal body temperature.

Proper monitoring of body temperature is essential when it comes to mastering ice baths for enhanced athletic performance. By regularly checking your body temperature, you can ensure a safe and effective ice bath session, prevent cold-related injuries, and optimize the benefits of this icy therapy. So, make sure to invest in reliable temperature monitoring tools and incorporate this crucial step into your ice bath routine for peak fitness.

Recognizing Signs of Cold Stress

In the pursuit of peak fitness and enhanced athletic performance, many fitness enthusiasts, sports people, gym goers, bodybuilders, athletes, and cross fit enthusiasts have turned to the power of icy therapy, particularly ice baths. These individuals understand the incredible benefits that cold exposure can have on their bodies, such as reduced inflammation, improved recovery times, and increased mental resilience. However, it is crucial to recognize the signs of cold stress to ensure the practice remains safe and effective.

Cold stress occurs when the body is exposed to extreme cold temperatures for an extended period. While ice baths are generally safe when done correctly, it is important to listen to your body and be aware of any warning signs that may indicate you are pushing your limits too far.

One of the most common signs of cold stress is shivering. Shivering is the body's natural response to cold temperatures, as it generates heat to help maintain a stable core temperature. However, if your shivering becomes uncontrollable or persists for an extended period, it may indicate that you are experiencing excessive cold stress.

Another sign to be mindful of is numbness or tingling in your extremities. When exposed to cold temperatures, blood vessels constrict, reducing blood ow to the extremities to protect the vital organs. If you notice persistent numbness or tingling in your hands, feet, or other body parts, it could be a sign that you need to exit the ice bath and warm up.

Additionally, pay attention to any changes in your skin color. Prolonged exposure to extreme cold can cause the skin to turn pale or even bluish in color, indicating poor blood circulation. If you notice such changes, it is crucial to exit the ice bath immediately and take steps to warm up.

Feeling excessively tired or fatigued during or after an ice bath is another sign of cold stress. While it is normal to feel a bit tired after a challenging session, if you find that your fatigue is overwhelming or persists for an extended period, it may indicate that you need to scale back your cold exposure and allow your body more time to recover.

Recognizing the signs of cold stress is essential for maintaining a safe and effective icy therapy routine. By being aware of your body's responses and taking appropriate action when necessary, you can continue to reap the incredible benefits of ice baths while minimizing the risk of injury or overexposure. Remember, icy resilience is about finding the balance between pushing your limits and listening to your body's needs.

Avoiding Overexposure and Hypothermia

When it comes to mastering the art of ice baths for peak fitness, it is crucial to understand the importance of avoiding overexposure and hypothermia. While ice baths offer numerous benefits for enhancing athletic performance, it is essential to practice them safely and responsibly. In this subchapter, we will delve into the strategies and precautions that fitness enthusiasts, sports people, gym-goers, bodybuilders, athletes, and cross fit enthusiasts should keep in mind to prevent overexposure and hypothermia during icy therapy sessions.

First and foremost, it is essential to establish a time limit for your ice baths. While pushing your limits is commendable, it is crucial to listen to your body and not exceed your physical capacity. Starting with shorter sessions, such as 1-2 minutes, and gradually increasing the duration over time is a prudent approach. This gradual progression allows your body to adapt to the cold temperatures and minimizes the risk of overexposure.

Monitoring your body temperature during an ice bath is another vital aspect of avoiding overexposure and hypothermia. Utilize a reliable thermometer to check your body temperature before, during, and after each session. If you notice that your body temperature drops below 95 degrees Fahrenheit (35 degrees Celsius), it is time to end the session immediately. This precautionary measure ensures that you do not subject your body to excessive cold stress.

Proper insulation is also crucial when engaging in icy therapy. Wearing a neoprene cap and gloves can help retain body heat and prevent excessive heat loss from your extremities. Additionally, consider using insulated mats or towels to sit on during the ice bath, as they act as a barrier between your body and the cold surface, further reducing the risk of hypothermia.

Lastly, always have a trained professional or a trusted partner present during your ice bath sessions. They can monitor your well-being, keep track of time, and assist you in case of any emergencies. Remember, safety should always be the top priority.

By following these guidelines and maintaining a responsible approach towards ice baths, you can reap the benefits of icy therapy without compromising your health. Overexposure and hypothermia are genuine risks, but with the right precautions, you can ensure a safe and effective ice bath experience.

Stay tuned for the next chapter, where we will explore the post-ice bath recovery techniques that will help you maximize the benefits of this powerful tool for enhancing athletic performance.

Chapter 8

Integrating Ice Baths into Your Fitness Routine

"Forget inspiration. Habit is more dependable. Habit
will sustain you whether you're inspired or not"

Octavia Butler

Frequency and Timing of Ice Baths

ONE OF THE MOST crucial aspects of mastering ice baths
for enhanced athletic performance is understanding the
frequency and timing at which they should be incorporated
into your training regimen. Ice baths, also known as cold-water
immersion therapy, have gained significant popularity among fitness

enthusiasts, sports people, gym-goers, bodybuilders, athletes, and cross-fit enthusiasts due to their numerous benefits on the body and mind.

When it comes to frequency, the key is to strike a balance. Ice baths should not be overused, as excessive exposure to cold temperatures can potentially have adverse eIects on the body. On the other hand, too infrequent use may not yield the desired results. Generally, it is recommended to incorporate ice baths into your routine two to three times per week, depending on your individual needs and training intensity.

Timing is also important when it comes to ice baths. The ideal time to take an ice bath is within one to two hours after intense physical activity. This timing allows the body to cool down naturally and prevents any potential in ammation or soreness that may arise from vigorous exercise. By immersing yourself in cold water during this window, you enhance the recovery process and minimize muscle damage.

However, it is important to note that ice baths are not limited to post-workout recovery. They can also be utilized before a workout as a means of preparing the body for physical exertion. Taking a short ice bath before a training session can help increase alertness, reduce fatigue, and improve overall performance. This pre-workout cold therapy stimulates the body's circulation and primes the muscles for optimal function.

Moreover, the duration of an ice bath is another factor to consider. While there is no set time frame that works for everyone, a typical ice bath session should last between 10 to 15 minutes. It is crucial to listen to your body and gradually build up your tolerance to the cold temperature. Starting with shorter durations and gradually increasing the time will help prevent any potential shock to the system.

In conclusion, mastering the art of ice baths for peak fitness requires an understanding of the frequency and timing at which they should be incorporated into your training routine. By striking a balance between not overusing or underutilizing ice baths, and by timing them correctly before or after intense physical activity, you can maximize their benefits on your athletic performance. Remember to start with shorter durations and gradually increase the time as your body adapts to the cold temperature. Embrace the power of icy resilience and unlock your full potential in the world of fitness and sports.

Ice Baths for Different Types of Athletes

Ice baths have become increasingly popular among athletes and fitness enthusiasts in recent years. This subchapter will explore how ice baths can benefit different types of athletes, including fitness enthusiasts, sports people, gym-goers, bodybuilders, athletes, and cross-fit enthusiasts.

For fitness enthusiasts and gym-goers, ice baths can provide a range of benefits. After an intense workout, muscles can become sore and inflamed. Ice baths help to reduce inflammation and promote muscle recovery by constricting blood vessels and flushing out waste products. This aids in reducing muscle soreness and fatigue, allowing fitness enthusiasts to recover more quickly and get back to their training routine.

Sports people, such as football players, basketball players, and runners, can also benefit from incorporating ice baths into their training regimen. Ice baths help to alleviate the stress and strain placed on the body during intense physical activity. By reducing inflammation and increasing blood circulation, ice baths can speed up the recovery process and prevent injuries. Additionally, ice baths can improve overall performance by enhancing muscle endurance and reducing muscle fatigue.

Bodybuilders, with their rigorous training routines and heavy lifting, can also benefit greatly from ice baths. By reducing inflammation and promoting muscle recovery, ice baths can help bodybuilders to achieve their desired physique. Ice baths can also aid in relieving muscle soreness, allowing bodybuilders to train more frequently and efficiently.

Athletes from various sports, such as swimmers, cyclists, and tennis players, can use ice baths to their advantage. These athletes often engage in repetitive and high-intensity movements, which can lead to muscle damage and fatigue. Ice baths can help to alleviate these symptoms by reducing inflammation and promoting muscle repair. This can ultimately improve their performance and prevent overuse injuries.

Lastly, cross-fit enthusiasts can incorporate ice baths into their training routine to enhance their overall fitness level. The intense nature of cross-fit workouts often leads to muscle soreness and fatigue. Ice baths aid in reducing these symptoms, allowing cross-fit enthusiasts to recover more quickly and continue pushing their limits.

In conclusion, ice baths can provide significant benefits for different types of athletes, including fitness enthusiasts, sports people, gym-goers, bodybuilders, athletes, and cross-fit enthusiasts. By reducing inflammation, promoting muscle recovery, and improving overall performance, ice baths have become an essential component of many athletes' training regimens. Whether you are looking to improve muscle recovery, prevent injuries, or enhance your overall fitness level, incorporating ice baths into your routine can help you achieve your goals faster and more effectively.

Long-Term Benefits and Maintenance

In the previous chapters, we have delved into the world of icy therapy and explored its numerous benefits for enhanced athletic performance. Now, let's take a closer look at the long-term advantages of incorporating ice baths into your fitness routine, as well as the essential aspects of maintenance to ensure optimal results.

One of the most significant long-term benefits of icy therapy is its ability to improve your overall recovery time. By subjecting your body to the extreme cold of an ice bath, you stimulate your blood vessels to constrict, reducing inflammation and swelling. This, in turn, accelerates the repair of damaged muscles and tissues, helping you recover faster from intense workouts or sports injuries. Regular ice baths can also aid in preventing muscle soreness and promote muscle growth, enabling you to push your limits during training sessions.

Moreover, icy therapy has been found to enhance the body's immune system. The exposure to cold temperatures activates the production of white blood cells, which are essential for fighting oI infections and diseases. By boosting your immune system, you can reduce the risk of falling ill and maintain consistent training schedules, leading to better performance over time.

To ensure you reap the long-term benefits of icy therapy, it is crucial to establish a proper maintenance routine. Firstly, always consult with a healthcare professional or a qualified trainer before incorporating ice baths into your fitness regimen, especially if you have any underlying health conditions. They can provide valuable guidance on the frequency and duration of your ice bath sessions based on your specific needs and goals.

Additionally, paying attention to the temperature and duration of your ice baths is essential. It is generally recommended to start with shorter sessions, gradually increasing the time as your body adapts to the cold. The ideal temperature for an ice bath ranges between 50 to 59 degrees Fahrenheit (10 to 15 degrees Celsius). However, every individual's tolerance level may vary, so always listen to your body and adjust accordingly.

Furthermore, remember to practice proper post-ice bath recovery techniques. These may include gentle stretching, foam rolling, or using heat therapy to promote blood ow and relaxation. Taking care of your body after an ice bath will enhance the overall benefits, ensuring that you are ready to tackle your next workout with renewed vigor.

Incorporating ice therapy into your fitness routine offers numerous long-term benefits for athletes, fitness enthusiasts, and sportspeople alike. From faster recovery times to a strengthened immune system, ice baths can give you the edge you need to excel in your chosen discipline. By following proper maintenance techniques and listening to your body, you can harness the power of icy resilience and take your athletic performance to new heights.

Chapter 9
Success Stories and Testimonials

Professional Athletes' Experiences with Ice Baths

ICE BATHS HAVE BECOME a popular recovery technique among professional athletes across various sports. These athletes, known for their dedication and commitment to peak performance, have incorporated ice baths into their training regimens to enhance their recovery and overall athletic performance. In this subchapter, we will explore the firsthand experiences of professional athletes with ice baths and how this practice has helped them achieve their fitness goals.

One common theme among professional athletes is the immediate relief and reduction in muscle soreness that ice baths provide. After intense training sessions or competitions, athletes often experience muscle inflammation and micro-tears, leading to soreness and discomfort. However, by immersing themselves in ice- cold water, these athletes have found that the cold temperature helps to constrict blood vessels, reducing inflammation and numbing the pain. This allows them to recover faster and get back to training with minimal downtime.

Moreover, ice baths have been praised for their ability to accelerate recovery by promoting circulation and flushing out metabolic waste products. The extreme cold stimulates vasoconstriction, causing blood vessels to constrict and then dilate upon exiting the ice bath. This process, known as vasodilation, brings fresh oxygenated blood to muscles, facilitating the removal of lactic acid and other waste products that can hinder performance. Athletes have reported feeling rejuvenated and energized after an ice bath, enabling them to perform at their best in subsequent training sessions or competitions.

Another significant benefit highlighted by professional athletes is the mental resilience developed through ice baths. Enduring the intense cold requires mental fortitude and discipline, traits that are essential for success in any athletic endeavour. By regularly subjecting themselves to the discomfort of ice baths, athletes strengthen their mental resolve and learn to push through physical and mental barriers. This mental resilience translates into improved performance on the field, court, or gym, as athletes are better equipped to handle adversity and stay focused during high-pressure situations.

In conclusion, professional athletes from various sports have attested to the positive impact of ice baths on their recovery and athletic performance. By reducing muscle soreness, promoting circulation, and fostering mental resilience, ice baths have become an integral part of their training routines. Whether you are a fitness enthusiast, bodybuilder, or cross-fit enthusiast, incorporating ice baths into your regimen can help you achieve your fitness goals and reach new heights in your athletic pursuits. Embrace the icy resilience and unlock your full potential with the mastery of ice baths.

Personal Testimonials from Ice Bath Enthusiasts

In this section, we delve into the personal testimonials of individuals who have embraced ice baths as an integral part of their fitness routines. These testimonials provide valuable insights into the transformative power of ice baths and how they have enhanced athletic performance and overall well-being.

1. Sarah, a dedicated gym-goer and bodybuilder, shares how incorporating ice baths into her recovery routine has been a game-changer. "After intense weightlifting sessions, I used to suffer from muscle soreness and fatigue. But ever since I started taking ice baths, my recovery time has significantly reduced. I feel rejuvenated and ready to hit the gym again the next day."

2. John, an avid runner, recounts how ice baths have improved his endurance and prevented injuries. "I used to struggle with shin splints and knee pain after long runs. But after implementing ice baths into my post-run routine, I've noticed a remarkable decrease in inflammation and discomfort. It's like my muscles and joints are getting a reset button after each session."

3. Laura, a professional athlete, shares how ice baths have

become an integral part of her training regimen. "Ice baths have been a game-changer for me. Not only do they help in reducing muscle soreness, but they also provide mental clarity and a sense of calmness. It's like a reset for both my body and mind, allowing me to perform at my best during competitions."

4. Mark, a crossfit enthusiast, reveals how ice baths have helped him push his limits and achieve new personal records. "Crossfit is all about pushing your boundaries, and ice baths have become an essential tool in my journey. They help me recover faster between intense workouts, allowing me to train harder and reach new levels of strength and performance."

These personal testimonials highlight the wide-ranging benefits of incorporating ice baths into your fitness routine. From accelerated recovery to improved endurance, mental clarity, and pushing physical limits, ice baths have the potential to revolutionize your athletic performance.

Whether you're a fitness enthusiast, sports person, gym-goer, bodybuilder, athlete, or part of the cross-fit community, embracing ice baths can unlock a whole new level of resilience and peak fitness. So why not take the plunge and join the ranks of these ice bath enthusiasts who have experienced firsthand the transformative power of icy therapy?

Inspiring Stories of Overcoming Challenges through Ice Baths

In the pursuit of peak fitness and athletic performance, individuals often encounter various physical and mental challenges. These obstacles can range from muscle soreness and fatigue to mental blocks and self- doubt. However, within the realm of icy therapy and the mastery of ice baths, remarkable stories of overcoming these challenges have emerged, providing inspiration and motivation for fitness enthusiasts, sportspeople, gym-goers, bodybuilders, athletes, and those engaged in cross fit.

"Icy Resilience: Mastering Ice Baths for Enhanced Athletic Performance" delves into the awe-inspiring tales of individuals who have harnessed the power of ice baths to push their limits, both physically and mentally. These real-life stories serve as powerful reminders that with determination, resilience, and the right tools, one can overcome any obstacle in their fitness journey.

One such story is that of Sarah, a determined athlete who suffered a severe knee injury during a marathon race. Devastated and faced with the possibility of never competing again, she turned to icy therapy as a means of rehabilitation. Through consistent ice bath sessions, Sarah not only managed to alleviate her pain but also discovered a newfound mental strength that helped her persevere through the grueling recovery process. Today, Sarah stands as a testament to the transformative power of ice baths, as she successfully completed her first triathlon post-injury.

Another inspiring account features Mark, a bodybuilder who struggled with muscle soreness and fatigue after intense training sessions. Despite his dedication to his craft, these physical challenges threatened to hinder his progress. However, after incorporating ice baths into his recovery routine, Mark noticed a significant improvement in his recovery time, enabling him to train more frequently and intensively. His commitment to icy therapy paid oI when he won his first bodybuilding competition, surpassing all expectations.

These stories, and many others like them, illustrate the incredible potential of ice baths to enhance athletic performance and overcome seemingly insurmountable challenges. This book provides a comprehensive guide to mastering the art of ice baths, offering practical tips, scientific insights, and inspiring anecdotes from individuals who have harnessed the power of cold therapy.

Whether you are an aspiring athlete, a fitness enthusiast, or someone seeking to push your limits, the inspiring stories within this subchapter will ignite your passion and remind you that with perseverance and the right mindset, you can conquer any challenge that comes your way. Embrace the power of icy resilience and unlock your true potential in the world of fitness and athletic performance.

Chapter 10

Taking Your Ice Bath Practice to the Next Level

"Successful people are always thinking about what they can do to move to the next level. Initiative is the drive to do it – to take the first step, and then the next step"

Maria Bartiromo

Advanced Techniques for Ice Baths

IN THE PURSUIT OF peak fitness and enhanced athletic performance, ice baths have emerged as a powerful tool for recovery and resilience. While the benefits of icing sore muscles and reducing inflammation are well- known, there are advanced techniques that can take your ice bath experience to the next level. In this part, we will explore some of these techniques and how they can be incorporated into your icy therapy routine.

1. Progressive Temperature Control: Rather than subjecting your body to extremely cold temperatures right away, consider gradually decreasing the temperature of the water over multiple sessions. This progressive approach allows your body to adapt and ultimately endure colder temperatures, maximizing the benefits of the ice bath.

2. Contrast Therapy: Alternating between hot and cold water can provide a more dynamic recovery experience. Start with a warm water soak, then switch to an ice bath for a few minutes. Repeat this cycle a few times to stimulate circulation and accelerate the recovery process.

3. Breathing Techniques: Deep breathing exercises can help you withstand the intense cold of an ice bath. Techniques like Wim Hof Method or controlled rhythmic breathing can help regulate your body's response to the cold, enabling you to stay in the ice bath for longer durations.

4. Active Movement: Rather than passively sitting in the ice bath, incorporate gentle exercises like leg raises or arm circles to engage your muscles. This active movement promotes blood ow and aids in flushing out metabolic waste products, expediting recovery.

5. Visualization and Mindfulness: Ice baths can be mentally challenging, but incorporating visualization

and mindfulness techniques can help you overcome the discomfort. Focus on positive imagery or practice mindfulness meditation to distract your mind from the cold and maintain a calm state throughout the session.

6. Gradual Exposure: If you are new to ice baths, start with shorter durations and gradually increase the time as your body adapts. Pushing your limits too soon can lead to discomfort or even shock. Remember, the goal is to build resilience over time, not to push yourself to the brink.

By implementing these advanced techniques, you can elevate your ice baths from a simple recovery practice to a transformative experience for your body and mind. Whether you are a fitness enthusiast, athlete, or gym-goer, mastering the art of ice baths will undoubtedly enhance your athletic performance and overall well-being. Embrace the cold, push your limits, and unlock the full potential of icy resilience.

Experimenting with Temperature Variations

One of the key aspects of mastering ice baths for enhanced athletic performance is understanding the importance of temperature variations. In this subchapter, we will delve into the various ways you can experiment with temperature variations to maximize the benefits of icy therapy.

Temperature variations play a crucial role in ice baths as they stimulate different physiological responses in the body. By manipulating the temperature of the water, you can target specific benefits and improve your overall fitness and recovery.

One technique you can try is the contrast bath method. This involves alternating between hot and cold water to promote blood circulation and reduce muscle soreness. Start by immersing yourself in a cold bath for a few minutes, then switch to a hot bath for an equal amount of time. Repeat this cycle multiple times to reap the rewards of increased blood flow and enhanced recovery.

Another temperature variation technique is progressive cooling. Begin with a comfortably warm bath and gradually add ice or cold water to decrease the temperature. This gradual cooling process allows your body to adapt to the cold and prevents shock to your system. Progressive cooling is ideal for beginners or those who are sensitive to extreme cold temperatures.

For those seeking a more intense experience, extreme temperature variations can be incorporated. Alternate between immersing yourself in an ice-cold bath and a hot bath or sauna. This extreme contrast challenges your body's resilience and can contribute to improved cardiovascular health and enhanced endurance.

It's important to note that experimenting with temperature variations should be done gradually and with caution. Listen to your body and adjust the intensity according to your comfort level. It's always recommended to consult with a professional or experienced ice bath practitioner before attempting extreme temperature variations.

By experimenting with temperature variations, you can unlock the full potential of icy therapy for peak fitness. Whether you're a fitness enthusiast, athlete, or bodybuilder, incorporating temperature variations into your ice bath routine can accelerate your recovery, reduce post-workout soreness, and enhance your overall athletic performance.

Remember, mastering the art of ice baths requires dedication and perseverance. Embrace the challenges and push your limits to experience the incredible benefits that icy therapy has to offer. Stay cool, stay resilient, and continue your journey towards peak fitness with temperature variations.

Pushing Your Limits and Embracing Discomfort

In the pursuit of peak fitness and enhanced athletic performance, it is crucial to challenge yourself beyond your comfort zone. This section will delve into the concept of pushing your limits and embracing discomfort, with a focus on the powerful tool of icy therapy - mastering the art of ice baths.

Fitness enthusiasts, sportspeople, gym-goers, bodybuilders, athletes, and CrossFit enthusiasts, this chapter is dedicated to you. Whether you are a professional athlete or someone striving to improve your fitness level, understanding the importance of pushing your limits and embracing discomfort is paramount.

When it comes to achieving extraordinary results, stepping outside your comfort zone is essential. Pushing your limits means pushing beyond what you think is possible, challenging your body and mind to adapt and grow. Embracing discomfort is about willingly subjecting yourself to challenging situations, knowing that they will ultimately lead to personal growth and improved performance.

One of the most effective ways to push your limits and embrace discomfort is through icy therapy, specifically ice baths. Ice baths have been used for centuries to aid in recovery, reduce inflammation, and boost performance. By subjecting your body to the shock of cold water, you force it to adapt and become more resilient.

Not only do ice baths provide physical benefits, but they also develop mental fortitude. Stepping into freezing water can be an incredibly uncomfortable experience, but it teaches you to stay calm in the face of adversity. This mental toughness translates into all areas of life, allowing you to overcome challenges with a newfound strength.

By mastering the art of ice baths, you will unlock a powerful tool for achieving peak fitness and athletic performance. So, let us embark on this journey together, embracing discomfort and pushing our limits to reach new heights of resilience and success.

Chapter 11
Conclusion

"Push yourself to do more and to experience more. Harness your energy to start expanding your dreams. Yes, expand your dreams. Don't accept a life of mediocrity when you hold such infinite potential within the fortress of your mind. Dare to tap into your greatness"

Robin Sharma

Recap of Key Takeaways

THROUGHOUT "ICY RESILIENCE" WE have explored the incredible benefits of incorporating ice baths into your fitness routine. Whether you are a fitness enthusiast, sports person, gym-goer, bodybuilder, athlete, or cross-fit enthusiast, the practice of icy therapy can help you achieve peak fitness levels and enhance your overall performance.

One key takeaway from this book is that ice baths can significantly reduce inflammation and promote muscle recovery. By subjecting your body to cold temperatures, you activate a process called vasoconstriction, which constricts blood vessels and reduces swelling. This accelerates the removal of waste products and brings fresh, oxygenated blood to the muscles, facilitating faster healing and reducing soreness.

Another important takeaway is that ice baths can improve cardiovascular health and endurance. When exposed to cold temperatures, your body works harder to maintain its core temperature, leading to an increase in heart rate and improved circulation. Regularly engaging in icy therapy can enhance your cardiovascular capacity, allowing you to endure longer and more intense workouts.

Furthermore, ice baths have been shown to boost mental resilience and improve mental clarity. The shock of cold water triggers the release of endorphins, which are natural mood elevators. This can help combat stress, anxiety, and depression, allowing you to approach your fitness goals with a positive mindset and unwavering determination.

To maximize the benefits of icy therapy, it is crucial to follow a few key guidelines. Firstly, always start with shorter durations and gradually increase the time spent in the ice bath. This will allow your body to adapt and avoid any potential risks. Additionally, it is important to maintain proper hydration before and after each session, as this aids in the recovery process.

In conclusion, "Icy Resilience" has provided invaluable insights into the world of icy therapy. By incorporating ice baths into your fitness routine, you can experience reduced inflammation, improved muscle recovery, enhanced cardiovascular health, and increased mental resilience. Embrace the power of icy therapy, and unlock your true athletic potential.

Embracing the Power of Ice Baths

Ice baths, once considered a secret weapon of elite athletes, are now gaining popularity among fitness enthusiasts, sportspeople, gym-goers, bodybuilders, athletes, and CrossFit enthusiasts alike. In the subchapter titled "Embracing the Power of Ice Baths" from the book "Icy Resilience: Mastering Ice Baths for Enhanced Athletic Performance," we dive into the transformative benefits of this icy therapy. Whether you're a professional athlete or a weekend warrior, understanding the power of ice baths can take your fitness journey to new heights.

Ice baths, also known as cold-water immersion therapy, involve submerging your body in icy water for a specific duration. While the initial shock of the cold can be intimidating, the rewards are worth it. By subjecting your body to such extreme temperatures, you can tap into a range of physiological and psychological advantages.

First and foremost, ice baths are known to speed up recovery post-workout. The cold water triggers vasoconstriction, causing blood vessels to constrict and reduce inflammation. As a result, muscle soreness and swelling are alleviated, allowing for faster recovery and reduced downtime between training sessions.

Furthermore, ice baths enhance athletic performance. Regular cold-water immersion has been shown to increase endurance, improve cardiovascular health, and boost overall strength and stamina. By regularly exposing yourself to the icy water, your body adapts to the stress, becoming more resilient and better equipped to handle physical exertion.

Beyond the physical benefits, ice baths also have a profound impact on mental well-being. The shock of cold water stimulates the release of endorphins, providing a natural mood boost and reducing stress and anxiety. Additionally, the cold exposure trains your mind to embrace discomfort, fostering mental toughness and resilience that can be applied to various aspects of life.

While ice baths offer numerous advantages, it's important to approach them with caution. Proper technique, duration, and temperature are key factors in harnessing their power safely and effectively. "Icy Resilience: Mastering Ice Baths for Enhanced Athletic Performance" provides expert guidance on the art of ice baths, ensuring you maximize the benefits while avoiding potential pitfalls.

Whether you're seeking to accelerate recovery, improve performance, or enhance your mental fortitude, embracing the power of ice baths is a game-changer. By incorporating this powerful tool into your fitness regimen, you'll unlock a world of physical and mental resilience, propelling you towards peak fitness and athletic excellence.

Final Words of Encouragement

Congratulations! You have made it. It's been quite a journey, hasn't it? You've learned about the incredible benefits of icy therapy and how it can take your fitness to new heights. Now, as we wrap up this book, we want to leave you with some final words of encouragement to inspire and motivate you on your path to peak fitness.

First and foremost, we want to remind you that you are capable of more than you can imagine. The mere fact that you have embarked on this icy therapy journey demonstrates your dedication to pushing the boundaries of your physical and mental capabilities. Embrace the discomfort, embrace the challenge, and know that every ice bath is an opportunity for growth.

Remember, progress is not always linear. There will be days when you feel strong and invincible, and there will be days when you struggle to find the motivation to step into that ice-filled tub. On those tough days, draw inspiration from your fellow fitness enthusiasts, sportspeople, gym-goers, bodybuilders, athletes, and CrossFit enthusiasts. Surround yourself with a community that understands the power of icy resilience and shares your passion for pushing limits.

In moments of doubt, remind yourself of the incredible benefits that icy therapy offers. Think about how it enhances your athletic performance, accelerates recovery, boosts your immune system, and improves your mental toughness. Re ect on the progress you have already made and let that fuel your determination to keep going.

Lastly, always prioritize self-care and listen to your body. While icy therapy can be an incredible tool, it's essential to find the right balance for your individual needs. Pay attention to any warning signs of overtraining or burnout and adjust your routine accordingly. Remember that rest and recovery are just as vital for your overall performance as the intense training sessions.

As you close this chapter of your icy therapy journey, we hope you feel inspired, motivated, and armed with the knowledge and tools to continue mastering the art of ice baths for peak fitness. Embrace the discomfort, embrace the challenge, and never stop striving for greatness. You have the power to become the best version of yourself. Keep pushing, keep growing, and continue to embrace icy resilience on your path to athletic excellence.

CHALLENGE. CHANGE. CHAMPION

Chapter 12

FAQs and Troubleshooting

"The will to win, the desire to succeed. The urge to reach your full potential – these are the keys that will unlock the door to personal excellence"

Confucius

Common Questions about Ice Baths

AS A FITNESS ENTHUSIAST, athlete, or someone interested in peak fitness, you may have heard about the benefits of ice baths for enhancing athletic performance. However, you may still have some questions about this icy therapy. In this subchapter, we will address some of the most common questions about ice baths and provide you with the answers you need to begin mastering the art of ice baths for peak fitness.

What is an ice bath, and how does it work?

An ice bath is a therapeutic practice that involves immersing your body in cold water, typically between 50 to 59 degrees Fahrenheit (10 to 15 degrees Celsius). The cold temperature constricts blood vessels and reduces inflammation, helping to relieve muscle soreness and speed up recovery.

How long should I stay in an ice bath?

The recommended duration for an ice bath is typically between 10 to 15 minutes. However, beginners may start with shorter durations, gradually increasing the time as they become more accustomed to the cold.

Can I use ice packs instead of immersing my whole body?

While ice packs can provide localized relief, immersing your whole body in an ice bath offers numerous benefits. It promotes overall muscle recovery, improves circulation, and boosts the release of endorphins.

When should I take an ice bath?

Ice baths are most effective when taken immediately after intense physical activity. This helps minimize muscle damage, reduce inflammation, and enhance recovery.

Are ice baths safe?

When done correctly, ice baths are generally safe. However, it's important to listen to your body and not push yourself beyond your limits. If you have any pre-existing medical conditions, it is advisable to consult with a healthcare professional before incorporating ice baths into your routine.

Can I take an ice bath every day?

While daily ice baths can be beneficial for some athletes, it's important to give your body time to recover. Starting with 2-3 ice baths per week and gradually increasing the frequency as your body adapts is a good approach.

Remember, mastering the art of ice baths requires patience and consistency. It is essential to listen to your body, gradually increase the duration and frequency, and seek guidance from a qualified professional if needed. By incorporating ice baths into your fitness routine, you can experience enhanced athletic performance, reduced muscle soreness, and accelerated recovery. So take the plunge and embrace the power of icy resilience!

Addressing Concerns and Misconceptions

In our quest for peak fitness and enhanced athletic performance, it is natural for us to explore every possible avenue. One such avenue that has gained considerable attention in recent years is the practice of ice baths. However, it is not uncommon for fitness enthusiasts, sportspeople, gym-goers, bodybuilders, athletes, and

CrossFit enthusiasts to have concerns and misconceptions about this form of therapy. In this subchapter, we will address those concerns and debunk any myths surrounding ice baths, helping you make an informed decision.

One of the most common concerns is the fear of hypothermia or frostbite. It is important to note that ice baths are not intended to freeze your body. Instead, they provide a controlled exposure to cold temperatures, typically ranging from 10 to 15 degrees Celsius. This temperature range is well-tolerated by the human body and does not pose a risk of frostbite or hypothermia when practiced correctly.

Another misconception is that ice baths are only beneficial for professional athletes or extreme fitness enthusiasts. On the contrary, ice baths can be beneficial for individuals at all fitness levels. Whether you are a weekend warrior, gym-goer, or someone recovering from an injury, incorporating ice baths into your routine can help reduce inflammation, enhance recovery, and improve overall performance.

Some individuals worry that ice baths may hinder muscle gains or negatively impact their training progress. However, research suggests that ice baths can actually complement your training regimen. By reducing inflammation and promoting faster recovery, ice baths can help you train more frequently and with higher intensity, ultimately leading to greater gains in strength and endurance.

There is also a misconception that ice baths are incredibly uncomfortable or even painful. While it is true that ice baths can be initially shocking to the system, your body will adapt to the cold over time. With regular practice, you will find that the discomfort diminishes, and you may even begin to enjoy the invigorating sensation provided by the cold immersion.

In conclusion, it is important to address concerns and misconceptions surrounding ice baths to fully understand their potential benefits. Ice baths are a safe and effective tool for enhancing athletic performance, aiding recovery, and promoting overall well-being. Whether you are a fitness enthusiast, sports person, gym-goer, bodybuilder, athlete, or CrossFit enthusiast, incorporating ice baths into your routine can take your fitness journey to new heights. So embrace the cold, master the art of ice baths, and unlock your icy resilience!

Troubleshooting Tips for Effective Ice Bath Sessions

In this subchapter, we will delve into troubleshooting tips for effective ice bath sessions. Ice baths are a powerful tool for enhancing athletic performance and recovery. However, to maximize their benefits, it is essential to ensure that you are conducting your ice bath sessions correctly. This section aims to address common problems and provide practical solutions for fitness enthusiasts, sportspeople, gym-goers, bodybuilders, athletes, and CrossFit enthusiasts who want to master the art of ice baths for peak fitness.

Maintaining the Optimal Temperature:

One of the key challenges faced during ice bath sessions is maintaining the ideal temperature. To tackle this issue, start by using a reliable thermometer to measure the water temperature accurately. Aim for a range of 50-59°F (10-15°C) for optimal results. If the temperature drops below this range, consider adding more ice or cold water to maintain the desired temperature throughout the session.

Overcoming Discomfort:

Ice baths can be uncomfortable, especially for beginners. To make the experience more bearable, focus on deep breathing and mental relaxation techniques. Practice mindfulness and visualize the benefits of the ice bath, such as reduced inflammation and improved recovery. Gradually increase the duration of your sessions to build resilience over time.

Dealing with Numbness and Tingling Sensations:

Numbness and tingling sensations are common during ice baths. However, if these sensations become too intense or painful, it is important to take immediate action. Ensure that you are not spending excessive time in the ice bath, as prolonged exposure can lead to frostbite or other complications. If the discomfort persists, consult with a healthcare professional.

Avoiding Shivering:

Shivering can interfere with the effectiveness of your ice bath session. To prevent shivering, try to warm up your body before entering the ice bath. Engage in light exercise or take a warm shower to increase your body temperature. Additionally, consider using a warm towel or blanket to cover your upper body during the session, focusing on keeping your core warm.

Hydration and Nutrition:

Proper hydration and nutrition play a vital role in optimizing the benefits of ice baths. Ensure that you are well-hydrated before and after your session. Replenish your body with electrolytes and nutrients by consuming a balanced meal or a recovery drink after the ice bath. This will aid in muscle recovery and reduce the risk of dehydration.

Conclusion:

By implementing these troubleshooting tips, you can enhance the effectiveness of your ice bath sessions and reap the maximum benefits for your athletic performance and recovery. Remember, mastering the art of ice baths requires patience, consistency, and a willingness to adapt to individual needs and preferences. Stay resilient, push your limits, and embrace the cold for peak fitness!

Also By CK

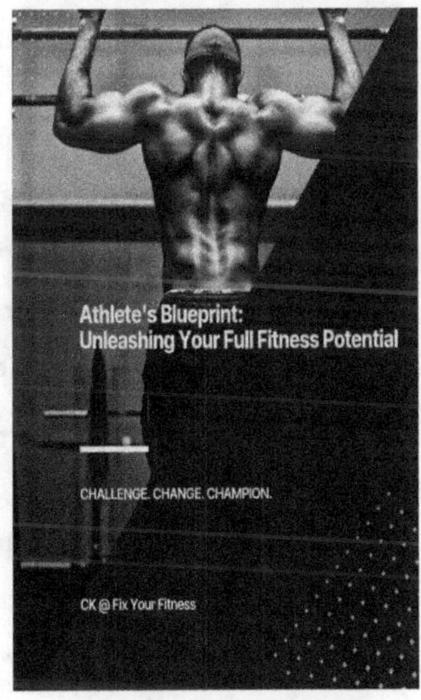

Athlete's Blueprint:

Unleashing Your Full Fitness Potential

About the Author

Hello, fitness enthusiasts!

Welcome to "Fix Your Fitness". Commonly known as 'CK', he's an expert in personal training, with a wealth of experience and a steadfast dedication to evidence-based fitness methodologies. His life's work has been in the realm of fitness, driven by a firm belief in the transformative power of physical and mental discipline.

Why this dedication? CK is a firm believer in the power of transformation – not merely in terms of physical appearance or strength, but more importantly, in mindset, determination, and spirit. He understands that everyone possesses an innate strength and potential, which sometimes requires a little guidance to fully realize.

His professional journey in the fitness industry has been both enlightening and deeply rewarding. CK has witnessed the incredible transformations of numerous individuals who have taken up the challenge to better themselves, addressing their weaknesses and building resilience. His philosophy is simple yet profound: anyone can be a champion in their own right. For him, fitness is not about winning races or lifting the heaviest weights, but about conquering personal challenges and growing stronger, wiser, and more resilient.

At "Fix Your Fitness", CK merges time-tested training techniques with cutting-edge scientific research. His approach is grounded in the science of the human body, ensuring that each fitness journey is effective, efficient, and safe. He eschews fads and quick fixes in favor of real, sustainable results.

In addition to his training and coaching, CK runs his own blog at fix-your-fitness.com. The blog is a rich resource of articles and eBooks covering all facets of fitness and health-related issues. It's a platform where he shares his extensive knowledge and insights, offering advice, tips, and in-depth information on various aspects of fitness, from workout routines to nutrition, mental health, and holistic wellness.

Whether you're at the start of your fitness journey or seeking to enhance and optimize your regimen, CK is there to guide, support, and motivate you toward your goals. 'Challenge. Change. Champion.' This mantra encapsulates his commitment to each individual's fitness journey, promising a transformative experience for all who join him. Let's embark on this journey together.

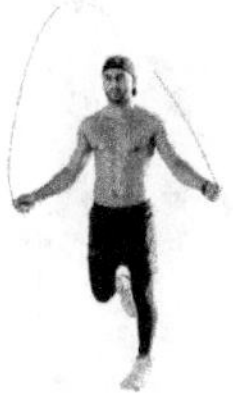

a   amazon.com/author/ck_fix-your-fitness

y   https://twitter.com/fixyourfitness1